SERIES TITLE
The Temple Building Workshops Presents

I0410005

BOOK TITLE
Healing Through Nature's Eyes

VOLUME TITLES
Vol. 1 – **Revealing the Mysteries of Natural Healing**
Vol. 2 – **Learning Your Wellness Language**
Vol. 3 – **Eloquence in Nature's Healing Language**

BOOK DESCRIPTION

Nature speaks a lovely, exotic language that reveals all of the information needed to understand its healing power and to awaken your body's natural healing abilities. It is the holistic language of harmony and balance. Once you attune yourself to your own personal wellness language, the path to health and wellness becomes clear.

This course series is designed to awaken you to the fact that you have a wellness language all your own that offers priceless guidance in your quest for natural healing. It is also my desire that you would become fluent in this language and learn how best to respond, and that any confusion surrounding the use of natural and alternative measures can be eliminated, leaving you with a new respect and appreciation for holistic, natural health.

Volume 1 - Revealing the Mysteries of Natural Healing

As sickness, disease or illness of any kind indicates an imbalance within, nature seeks to correct this imbalance by providing several healing dynamics which I refer to as natural healing guidelines.

Volume 1 introduces these guidelines found in nature that, when balanced in your daily life, will aid you in reaching optimal health and healing and explains how the use or neglect of these affect you holistically. Learn these, then complete the Health Balance Exercise. You might be surprised at the information revealed about your healthy balance and holistic wellness status!

Volume 2 – Learning Your Wellness Language

Nature communicates with you, and you subconsciously respond in your own unique language. However, most people never tune in on this most important conversation because it has been silenced by both internal and external distractions.

Volume 2 helps you to recognize the fact that messages are being sent and received within your totally holistic self, with nature, and that it's in your best interest to listen! It also shows how to interpret your personal language, and how best to respond. Understanding your personal wellness language is the key to knowing your health and wellness needs. It is our hope that this information will enable you to begin creating your personal, balanced healing regimen and begin to experience the natural healing you've been seeking.

Volume 3 – Eloquence in Nature's Healing Language

When you have become proficient in the healing language of nature, **Volume 3** teaches you to fine-tune your skills so that your immediate and accurate corrective response to any imbalance will become second nature. As you have no doubt discovered the unparalleled potential of these incredibly effective, natural health tools, your life should now be on track for reaching optimal wellness and a wonderful, holistic lifestyle that keeps you in sync with the healing balance of nature!

From regular exercising to juicing, consuming sufficient amounts of food and water and getting adequate sleep hours, to practicing vegetarianism, the information is endless, and it can really become overwhelming as you try to figure out what, when and how to juggle and balance these into your regular schedule. Well, help is available, and the time is now to begin your journey to natural, holistic health and wellness!

FOREWORD

Just think about it! We are not man-made constructions of metal and glass. We are wonderful, living, breathing creations, taken from the very substances of nature. When we eat plant-based foods, our body prepares this food to be assimilated through the process of digestion. During the course of digestion, the body absorbs nutrients that are required for the efficient functioning of our organs and the numerous metabolic processes that support and maintain our health and wellness.

At the first sign of attack by disease or illness, our defenses are set in motion, terminating any intruders and repairing any breaches. When you think about this fact, it makes perfect sense that, when given the proper nourishment and sustenance, while eliminating anything that will weaken or undermine health, the human body's ability to heal itself is fully and holistically fortified, supported and activated.

As you learn more about natural health, it is our hope that you will allow your spirit to connect with this holistic truth that is in harmony with nature and with God. Allow any seeds of hope to take root, blossom and produce the vibrant, natural healing lifestyle that you have been seeking, because it *is* available to you now!

Open your heart to envision the *Healing Through Nature's Eyes* series, in its beautiful simplicity, as your keys to natural health and healing. In Volume One,

Revealing the Mysteries of Natural Healing, nature's mysteries beautifully unfold to reveal the healing, strengthening effects these practices exert upon the human body.

Think of these guidelines in nature as a "good health" recipe. Our bodies require a balanced combination of materials to get healthy and stay healthy. All of these substances, which are abundant in our world, are found in nature, in the right forms, and in the right combinations for us.

When we put these guidelines into daily practice, we are taking advantage of the perfect recipe for optimal health. And like a recipe, we must include all of the necessary ingredients. Imagine what would happen if the bakery made a cake with butter, eggs, and milk, but left out the flour and the sugar! You'd probably end up with an omelet! Picture in your mind how all of the ingredients **work together** to give you the end results. What is your recipe, and what is the desired end result of your recipe?!

You can also think of the natural health guidelines as your care and usage instructions. When you make these health practices your regular habit, they serve to ensure that your body, mind, and spirit will each function as the Creator intended – efficiently, productively and without illnesses or diseases. It was God's plan that we would live vital, healthy, happy lives, and He made all the necessary provisions to ensure that we could do just that.

The God Connection

A whole and healthy God Connection is the cornerstone of your holistic health. A relationship with The Universal Mind that is based on faith, trust and love will prompt you to seek natural, holistic health – a healing of mind, body, and spirit – and that relationship will sustain and uplift you in your journey.

Maintain your connection with the Source of all strength, and you will find health and healing abundantly. Make spiritual communion a priority and you will find happiness and peace beyond your most vivid imagination!

"As I sit in quiet meditation, my soul is stilled and calmed. All clutter and chaos dims until it is silenced, and I feel a sense of divine peace and tranquility. I grow aware of my heart's opening, and my spirit soars in anticipation as once again, my ears become attuned to the voice of God"

Journal of My Spiritual Journey

Knowing God is not necessarily a 'church' thing, but is a very personal and intimate relationship with your God. Although the practice of attending organized worship services will generally add to your spiritual health, including others in your God Connection is not a requirement for you to achieve a healthy balance.

Your spirit is a vital part of your holistic being, and can become unbalanced just as easily as can your physical and mental self. This deepest, inner part of you, your spirit, must receive sufficient nourishment, nurturing and focused attention to attain this crucial, healthy balance and remain at your optimal healthy status.

Daily Activities for a Healthy Spirit
Recommendations:

1. **Focused Prayer**
   Make this a special, undivided period of time to talk with and listen to God
2. **Inspirational Readings**
   Read a daily devotional or other spiritual or inspirational material
3. **Praise & Worship**
   Openly express heartfelt gratitude in all things, whether done publicly or privately
4. **Spiritual Study**
   Research to gain spiritual insight and firmly establish your personal belief system. Remember that your inner beliefs are the key influences of your outer reality. Seek knowledge to better understand your spiritual needs
5. **Meditation**
   Although this is a separate focus, you can easily combine it with your God Connection period

Why is this important?

Meditation: A Healthy Mind & Emotions

Most of us encounter a daily storm of audible chaos and clutter, especially in this technological world of ours. There are so many distractions to detract from that which matters most. Then, consider the assault upon our minds by subliminal messages. Most of us are rarely aware that this attack is even taking place. One must wonder if there is some devious plan to keep us distanced from God – the Source of our every strength and power.

Meditation is a simple, alternative healing art that teaches one to quiet and focus the mind. It is a time to listen and connect. It teaches us stability, clarity, balance and is the path to enlightenment. This awesome practice goes hand-in-hand with prayer, and helps to strengthen our awareness of and connection to the Divine.

When we meditate, we learn to silence the mental chatter and become aware of the deeper thoughts and beliefs within our own mind – those mental/emotional elements that have an effect on every aspect of our lives. At this point, we must decide if these thoughts are positive or negative, healing or destructive, and determine what actions must take place to ensure movement towards healing and creativity.

Your mind forms the basis of who you are. Guard and protect it diligently!

When in prayer, I humbly share my daily story with the Divine. Then, in meditation, I sit quietly in earnest, joyful anticipation of God's message to me...
Journal of My Spiritual Journey

Meditation Styles

Guided Meditation
Motivational speakers often record powerful, appealing messages that if heeded, will enable you to erase negative mental chatter and replace it with positive beliefs and affirmations

Silent Meditation
Regular, daily periods of solitary silence are often sufficient for soothing the soul, and disciplining the mind. Silent meditation is particularly effective immediately after prayer, encouraging one to quietly listen to any divine messages from God

Meditation with Ambient Music
To help create a calming, healing environment for the listener, many guided meditations include ambient background music – very appealing to the meditating music lover

Chanting Meditation
Chanting meditations make use of Sanskrit mantras, and are often a part of Eastern religious practices. The chanted words or sounds have meanings that are believed to be helpful in strengthening the personal energy centers or Chakras

Daily Activities for A Healthy Mind & Emotions
<u>Recommendations</u>**:**

1. **Daily Meditation Practice** – Keeps your mind both alert and rested. Meditation promotes mental rejuvenation and clarity
   o Meditate from 10 minutes to 3 hours daily, incorporating a style that appeals to you (you may find several appealing)
   o Obtain recorded meditations from trusted sources. Avoid mind-controlling meditations that use hypnosis or subliminal messages

2. **Guard your Mind & Spirit** – Be mindful of those things that you allow to access your psyche. Keep it positive!
   o Determine the types of mental chatter you are creating
   o Utilize meditations and affirmations that focus on replacing all negatives with positives

3. **Cultivate Spiritual Fruit** – Love, gratitude, kindness, forgiveness, patience, faith, and joy all radiate high energetic vibrations and inspire mental/emotional awareness and enlightenment, acceptance and clarity
   o Make meditation a part of your God connections – set aside time to listen quietly

4. **Exercise the Mind** – Make time to actively engage in mind-strengthening activities
   o Both formal and self-education are excellent mind-exercising tools
   o Stimulate and strengthen your mind by studying the arts, math, history, the sciences and other positive, uplifting subjects
   o Read regularly
   o Learn something new and creative every day

5. **Remain True to Yourself** – Emotions are a normal part of who you are. They must be nurtured and balanced to stay healthy.
   o Develop habits that support self-awareness with honesty and integrity

(Seek professional Mental Health counseling or treatment as needed)

<u>**Why is this important?**</u>

Exercise & Recreation

Healthy Exercise:

- helps to bring the skeletal system into alignment and helps to corrects mild skeletal deformities
- helps to correct bowel irregularities by building and toning abdominal muscles
- helps to strengthen and tone the vital organs
- strengthen muscles that promote good posture, which promotes deep breathing and lung expansion
- helps to regulate and stabilize the heart rate
- increases and promotes a positive self-image and self esteem
- helps to correct obesity and helps to maintain a normal, healthy weight
- helps to regulate the appetite and stimulates the desire for healthful foods
- helps to eliminate excess physical and mental stress, decreases depression and promotes a sense of well-being
- helps to improve and correct poor circulation by stimulating the growth of new capillaries

Exercise is a good stressor that is needed to keep our bodies in balance. As we move towards attaining optimum health, we begin to view our regular exercise regimen as a relaxing, healthful activity to be anticipated rather than dreaded.

Establish an exercise routine that will grow with you. Begin with light exercise and increase the difficulty according to your ability. Our bodies do not require discomfort to achieve tone and strength. The key to experiencing the remarkable benefits of exercise is consistency. The human body was made to grow and strengthen with a balance of exercise, recreation, relaxation, and sleep. Be kind to yourself, especially in this area!

Many jobs requiring strenuous physical activity offer the extra advantage of combining work with exercise time, which is an excellent way to fulfill your daily or weekly exercise requirements. However, physical labor jobs represent only a very small percentage of employment positions. Many of us, especially those with sedentary jobs, must purposely schedule time to engage in regular physical exercise and recreation to maintain our healthy balance.

Imparting strength and tone to the muscles and internal organs, expanding and strengthening the lungs through deep breathing, and stress relief are several, wonderful benefits of **Physical Exercise**. Regular, physical exercise also helps to improve digestion, and promotes more restful sleep habits. Plus, you will gain immense, personal satisfaction when you display a strong, muscular, healthy physique!

Recreation has many of the same benefits as regular exercising, but with the added elements of fun and social interactions. Play time with family and friends has very positive effects on your holistic health, imparting a sense of well-being and happiness. Having audacious fun acts as a pressure release valve, and allows you to truly relax and breathe.

Daily Activities for Healthful Exercising

<u>Recommendations</u>:

1. **Begin slowly** – Even if you feel that you can lift more, run farther, or exercise longer, begin at or below your abilities, especially if it's been a while since you've exercised. Gradually increase your exercise weights, times and reps as you are able to do so without injury.

2. **Become creative in making your daily activities a part of your exercise regimen** – Do a few foot and ankle exercises while sitting; Do squats while talking on the phone or watching TV; put extra focus on any lifting, bending, stretching, contracting of muscles, etc. that you might do in a day's work and make it count towards your daily exercise regimen.

3. **Pain is NOT gain!** – A bit of soreness from exercising is normal, particularly if you're new to it, and you might occasionally feel a muscle burn sensation during your workout when flexing and contracting unused muscles. But if any exercise causes you pain, stop doing it immediately, and enlist the help of a personal trainer! Exercising is a natural, healthful and enjoyable activity that should feel as normal to your body as breathing once it becomes your regular habit.

4. **Beginners** – Exercise 2-3 times per week for 30 minutes; **Advanced** – Exercise 3-5 times per week for 1 hr. or more. **Experts** – at your own discretion.

5. **Become Knowledgeable about Exercising** – Invest in exercise DVDs, online instructions, a fitness club or a reputable personal trainer to learn what exercises are best for you. Read books and articles on exercises and equipment, dietary needs for physical fitness, and any related topics that will help you to gain usable knowledge.

6. **Walking** in the fresh, open air is still the best all-around exercise. It has positive benefits on your muscle tone, your heart rate and circulation, your weight, your breathing, your mental health – and walking is still a FREE activity!

<u>Why is this important?</u>

Daily Activities for Healthy Recreation
<u>Recommendations</u>:

1. **Learn to have unabashed fun!** – It is vital to release the tensions and stresses that build up, and just play. Plan a fun period for at least 1 hour every day

2. **Join a Recreation Center** – Peruse the yearly schedule of seasonal activities that are sponsored by the center. Sign up for one event per year (or more as it suits you)

3. **Include Recreation in your Family's Schedule** – Plan a monthly outing with your family and/or friends. Keep it simple but fun, relaxing and full of laughter!

4. **Remember the Feeling** – You may be tired after a weekend of hiking, but enjoy the satisfaction, relaxation, and sense of fulfillment you experience after each recreational event!

5. **Plan other activities of your choice** – Be Creative. The list is endless!

<u>Why is this important?</u>

Relaxation & Restful Sleep

Relaxation

What is the difference between rest and sleep?

Rest is defined as the act or state of ceasing from work, activity, or motion: quiet. – Peace, ease or refreshment as a consequence of sleep or the cessation of an activity.

Sleep is defined as a natural, periodically recurring physiological state of rest marked by relative physical and nervous inactivity, unconsciousness, and lessened responsiveness to external stimuli.

We may therefore conclude that rest can lead to sleep, but is not necessarily a state of unconsciousness. We may rest without sleeping, or sleep without resting. But the ideal state of being is to have restful sleep, where all is peaceful and the body is fully relaxed, all activity has ceased, and the body can start the repair/rejuvenation process.

In today's world, everything is rush-rush, and many people feel that if you want to succeed in life, there is no time for resting or sleeping. Consequently, heart attacks, strokes, stomach ulcers, indigestion (esophageal reflux), panic/anxiety attacks, and other stress-related illnesses are on the rise. Additionally, pharmaceutical companies are earning exorbitant amounts of money for drugs prescribed to treat these illnesses when nature already contains instructions and solutions that would erase all of these problems.

If you have a high-stress occupation, relaxation becomes a vital requirement for health and life. Think of relaxation as a pressure release valve – which can be extremely important in helping to prevent serious life-threatening conditions such as stroke or heart attack. Even if your job is not 'high-stress', you still need relaxation time to unwind from your day-to-day labor.

Relaxation allows a respite from physical peak performance, thus your body slows and begins to function efficiently while requiring only minimal resources to do so. It's a bit like down-shifting from 4th to 1st gear. During your relaxation period, your body can focus any newly available energy on minor repairs and maintenance. Engaging in relaxing activities is also a great way for you to flow into a restful night's sleep where your body's internal repair crews are in full force while still utilizing minimal energy.

Daily Activities for Relaxation

Recommendations:

1. **Learn relaxation techniques that you can add to your daily schedule**

2. **Begin each daily relaxation technique with this deep breathing exercise –**
   - Breathe in slowly and deeply through your nose for 5 seconds
   - Slowly exhale through pursed lips
   - Repeat 3 – 5 times, then continue with relaxation technique(s)

3. **Practice relaxation techniques that are effective and enjoyable**
   - Make your relaxation time something to look forward to; make it stress-free
   - Do your selected techniques at least 30 minutes to 1 hour every day
   - Engage in relaxation techniques that leave you feeling rested and refreshed
   - Use tools that enhance your relaxation experience

Relaxation Tools Suggestions:

Scented Candles

Listening to Soothing music

A Warm Oil Massage

Sipping Chamomile Tea

Sitting on the beach

Reading a good book

A Leisurely Stroll

Sitting in A Rocking Chair

Sitting on a Porch swing

Swaying in a Hammock

A Warm bath

Other Tools of your Choice

Why is this important?

Restful Sleep

Deep, uninterrupted sleep allows your body to rest thoroughly from the heavy work of your activities, and your body's daily functions and metabolic processes. This is also the perfect and much needed time for intense healing.

When a person suffers severe physical trauma, the expected outcome, short of death, is a comatose condition. This is the deepest type of unconscious sleep, and is also the body's emergency response to the trauma. The body recognizes any life-threatening condition and begins to minimize the regular daily energy usage of normal processes so that all available energy can be re-routed and focused on stabilizing the trauma situation.

Even without physical trauma, the same process of healing is at work while we sleep nightly. The body recognizes any damage sustained in the course of a day, and sets about to repair, restore, and revitalize us for the next new day of being awake, alert and alive.

Though the body is in a continual healing state, intense healing requires 'down' time, when there are no other pressing energy demands. If your nightly, deep sleep is interrupted, the intense healing period is halted as the body must prepare itself for awake-alert mode. Although a trip to the bathroom in the middle of the night is a false wake-up alarm, your body still assumes awake-alert status. It takes time to get back into a deep sleep mode, and the intense healing process will not resume until you do. Several interruptions throughout the night, or not getting to bed until late only to wake up extra early can mean that the healing period never happens. As you continue to miss out on deep sleep, the body begins to sustain damage faster than it can make repairs. Over time, this course will take its toll with the inevitable result: illness, disease, and eventually death.

The Solution: Every 24 hours, get sufficient, deep, restful sleep

Daily Activities for Restful Sleep
<u>Recommendations</u>:

1. The TBW rule is: if you are engaged in active labor for 8 hours per day, you should get 6 – 8 hours of sleep per day. Work 12 hours, sleep 10 – 12 hours a day (If you are ill, you will require additional sleep as your healing needs have increased – make allowances for this additional sleep time)
2. Practice relaxation techniques 30 minutes to 1 hour prior to bedtime
3. Wear loose-fitting, natural fiber clothing at bed-time. Avoid tight, binding, synthetic & stretch fabrics that can cinch and pinch
4. Finish meals at least 2 - 4 hours before bed-time to minimize chances of gastric discomfort or other sleep interruptions
5. Keep bedding clean and wrinkle-free
6. Turn off TVs, computers, cell phones and stereos before you drift off to sleep. Even though music can be relaxing, noises during your sleep time prevent you from entering the deep sleep phase, whether or not you are aware of it
7. Maintain a comfortable temperature in your sleeping area – no extremes; around 20 degrees below normal body temperature is acceptable.

<u>Why is this important?</u>

Fresh Air & Sunshine

History tells us that not too many years ago, women would keep their blinds closed to prevent the sunlight from fading the colors of their draperies, rugs, and furniture. However, the better health practice is to open the blinds and raise the windows because the sunshine killed harmful germs and bacteria that loved to cower in the dark, dank corners of homes. The fresh, pure air along with the wonderful sun rays help to freshen the home and promote a cheerful atmosphere.

How can air do anything for good health? It's just air!

Without air, we die. End of story

Not really the end of the story. Not only do we need air, that perfect mixture of oxygen, nitrogen, and lesser amounts of other chemical gases, but we need fresh, pure, clean air for our lungs to function properly and to stay healthy. Our lungs breathe in the oxygen from the air, and expel the carbon dioxide that we do not need. The oxygen is then processed by the lungs and distributed to the cells throughout our body.

A bit of interesting information I learned as an adult is that the air we breathe contains negatively and positively charged ions – electricity. That isn't the interesting part. What I found fascinating was that when we breathe *positively* charged air, we tend to feel adverse effects such as headaches, nasal obstruction, fatigue, dry throat, hoarseness, etc. However, breathing *negatively* charged ions not only promotes feelings of well-being, and reduces that stressed-out feeling, but has been shown to stabilize the respiratory rate and lower the blood pressure to normal, healthy levels!

So, how do we find out what kind of ions we are breathing? How can we find the good (negatively charged) ions?

Negatively charged ions are found in abundance near oceans, rivers, streams or waterfalls, in the mountains, and generally outdoors. As you might have guessed, enclosed buildings have mostly positively charged ions. And guess what else?! Not only do all electrical appliances and electronics gobble up the good ions and discharge positive ions, but so do people!

Bask in the sun. Take a walk through the trees. Listen to the sounds of the ocean. Climb a mountain. Just thinking about these activities gives us a sense of peace and well-being. I have decided that our Eternal Creator is awesome!

As children, my brother, sister and I were ready and eager to get outside about one hour after sunrise most summer mornings. We would play all day with the neighborhood kids in the southern sunshine, and except for toilet breaks, didn't return indoors until sunset. Many times, we even took lunch outside to eat with our friends, loving every minute of the sunshine, and we never suffered a single ill effect because of it!

Contrary to popular belief and opinion, it is very important to get plenty of daylight or sunshine daily, either directly or indirectly. Sunshine provides us with several vitamins, and is a wonderful germ fighter. Sunshine, Fresh Air and the great outdoors supply us with negative ions, which is widely known to have a positive effect on the blood pressure, the heart rate and your overall healing and sense of well-being. Sunbathe wisely, particularly if you have characteristics that predispose you to sun-related skin diseases

Fresh air is vital because without it, we die! Practice deep breathing throughout the day to expand the lungs, which helps to remove stale, oxygen-depleted air that has become trapped in the lower lobes as a result of shallow breathing. Fresh, oxygenated air replenishes the blood's oxygen supply, allowing sufficient quantities of oxygen to be transported to the vital organs

Activities for Enjoying Fresh Air & Sunshine
<u>Recommendations</u>:

1. **Step outside at least once a day** – rain or shine
   - **Being inside** for long periods exposes you to positive ions (the 'Bad' ions), which are released by electronics, appliances, electrical items and buildings or enclosed areas in general. These bad ions have negative effects on your heart rate, blood pressure, your stress level and sense of happiness & well-being.
   - **Being outside** allows you to breathe in the negative ions (the 'Good' ions), which are released by the sun, water, trees, mountains, grass, and just about everything in the natural outdoors. Negative ions promote and support natural health and healing.
   - **Sunshine** radiates a special warmth that reaches the soul, and has a healing effect on those who have been ill and confined inside.
   - **Being outside** in the sunshine just feels so good!

2. **Practice deep breathing outside whenever you can**
   - **Deep breathing** cleanses your lungs and imparts a sense of well-being. It helps to releases harmful stressors.
   - **Once outside**, inhale deeply. Stretch your arms and simply enjoy two more of God's healing natural gifts to us – sunshine & fresh air!

<u>**Why is this important?**</u>

Healthy Elimination

Defecation

Not enough emphasis is placed on normal, proper elimination of feces and urine. Yet again, it is vital for optimal health that you expel the waste matter produced by your body's metabolic processes. Regular bowel movements are necessary due to the fact that your intestines were designed for digestion and processing waste for evacuation – not for storage! Your bladder is designed to collect urine, but it does have a limited capacity, and must be emptied regularly since urine collection is a continuous process. Yet, many people give no thought to the vital necessity of waste removal, and therefore contain pounds of feces that should have been evacuated long ago, and over-extended bladders that begin to malfunction and fail!

Think about it. If you suffer from occasional or chronic constipation, compare that to having trash and garbage piled up in your home, and no one ever removes it. Think of the terrible conditions you would have to endure if you did empty the trash, but the sanitation workers organized a strike! Imagine the rats and other vermin, roaches, decay, filth & stench, and ultimately illnesses and diseases of epidemic proportions that would occur! This is similar to what goes on in your colon when you do not have regular elimination habits, including the decay, filth & stench, rats and other vermin of a different nature. Constipation is the perfect environment for a multitude of preventable illnesses and disease conditions. Remember that trash is constantly decaying no matter where it is. Rot and decay produce foul, unpleasant smells that attract those creatures that were designed for waste removal!

Urination

Then, there is the matter of urination – another subject that people generally do not want to discuss. The healthy kidneys create urine continually, and the ureters route urine from the kidneys to the bladder for collection.

We should urinate about every three to four hours, but at least once every eight hours. Because urine is simply liquid *waste* matter, it should be expelled regularly, rather than held in the bladder. Frequency in urination is often a sign or symptom of some type of illness or disease process in the body. Scanty urination is also a sign of the same.

Once the bladder reaches its capacity, a message is sent to you in the form of an urge to urinate, and when you receive that message, it is best to answer. If you are engaged in other activities at the time and decide to hold your urine, your body will comply – for a season. However, because your bladder was not designed as a permanent storage unit, routinely ignoring or delaying your need to urinate is unwise. This habit can and most often will result in several undesirable and debilitating, albeit preventable conditions to include, urinary retention, urinary incontinence, UTI, and others.

I have had patients who experienced the urge to urinate as often as every 30 minutes. Generally, this was the result of a disease process or surgical procedure, and not in any way a normal elimination pattern. Unless a person is drinking large amounts of liquid, or is receiving IV therapy, the bladder will not fill this rapidly. Attempting to "empty" an already empty bladder will cause the feeling of urgency to become more pronounced, and does not allow the urinary sphincter muscles to relax, thus creating one continuous negative cycle. Urinary frequency should be discouraged by using the three natural remedies I have listed below.

Three ways to remedy urinary frequency naturally:

1. **Kiegel exercises. Tighten the pelvic floor muscles and hold for 5 – 10 seconds, then release. Repeat this 5 to 10 times**
2. **Schedule your bathroom breaks for every 3 – 4 hours. If you feel a strong urinary urge, use the Kiegel exercises**
3. **There are herbs that are helpful for urinary frequency. It should be first determined that urinary frequency is not the result of another condition which might require medical attention.**

Basically, establishing regular bowel and bladder evacuation habits can help you to prevent a few unwanted renal health concerns and does absolutely promote your optimal healthy balance.

Activities for Normal Elimination
Recommendations:

Bowel Movements should –
... occur once after each meal
... be equivalent to the distance from your wrist to your elbow
... be solidly formed but soft and buoyant
... not have a foul, toxic odor

A well-balanced vegetarian diet usually helps to brings about good colon health and regular bowel elimination habits. If you have trouble establishing regularity, try adding more fresh fruits and water to your day. Increase daily intake of naturally occurring roughage and fiber and avoid soft, mushy foods. For more information, contact your naturopathic consultant about utilizing juicing, raw vegetable and/or fruit diets and sources of natural dietary fiber as healthy ways to address constipation or other bowel concerns. Consider colonics* as a last resort option

*I discourage the use of colonics unless under extreme emergency conditions. Seek the advice and guidance of your Natural Health Practitioner when choosing this treatment option

Urination should –
... occur every 3-4 hours while awake
... be clear, yellow, wheat or amber colored
... not contain blood, sediment or other matter
... not have a foul, toxic odor
... have a strong, forceful flow

If you don't feel the urge to urinate this regularly, you may need to increase your water intake. Your health and wellness requires that you stay well hydrated for numerous reasons. If you have problems with leakage or retention, consult your naturopathic health practitioner for information on bowel and bladder training programs for holistic living

Why is this important?

Pure Water

Pure water hydrates cells and flushes impurities from the body, inside out. Water helps to liquefy mucus, which decreases its viscosity, making it easier to expel from the respiratory tract. In short, you can cough up the phlegm and rid yourself of colds and flu bugs better when you are sufficiently hydrated!

It keeps body fluids their proper consistency. This means that water hydrates your blood helping it to flow more smoothly through your veins – this could possibly lessen the likelihood of blood clots which can lead to even more serious health conditions. Your saliva, your tears, your urine, all of your body fluids become less sluggish and viscous when well hydrated, thus helping them to accomplish their tasks more easily and efficiently.

A warm bath cleanses away odor & disease-causing bacteria from the skin, and is a wonderful treatment for painful muscles and joints or other aches and pains. The benefits of water are just too numerous to list. Water is life!

For Internal Hydration
- Drink between 32 and 64 ounces of water daily
- Drink water whenever you are feeling thirsty

For External Cleansing
- Bathe daily for cleanliness
- Give a tepid or lukewarm bath to help reduce fevers

Water will cool a fever, it flushes impurities from the body, and it keeps our bodily fluids free flowing and mobile. Bathing is an essential health habit, as it rids the body of dust, dirt, pollution, mites & insects, bacteria and other antigens. Such a simple solution to so many ills.

Water is the one ingredient present in every area of our body. We can live a lot longer without food than we can without water, so we must conclude that water is vital to life!

- Cleanses the body both internally and externally
- Keeps cells hydrated which promotes normal cellular activities (repair, reproduction, etc.)
- Refreshes our entire being and is the very best thirst quencher
- Promotes the mobility of vital nutrients, vitamins and minerals throughout the body
- Helps to prevent constipation, kidney stones, and other unhealthy accumulations in the body
- Keeps the blood of a normal, free-flowing consistency
- Important in ridding the body of dangerous antigens – germs and bacteria, etc.
- The list goes on...

"Cleanliness is just an obsession with some people"

"Cleanliness is next to Godliness" Daddy would always say. Water is a natural cleanser. When a body has sufficient water, the systems function more efficiently. It cannot be stressed enough that water keeps body fluids the proper consistency, thus promoting good circulation. Lack of sufficient water in the body creates stagnation and sluggish movement of body matter and body fluids (blood, saliva, semen, mucus, urine, etc.), thus creating an ideal environment for disease habitation and reproduction.

External cleansing by bath or shower is wonderful for overall health. The skin protects our internal systems from attack by germs and bacteria and other possible environmental damage. As we walk and breathe in our polluted cities, ride on public transportation, or interact with others, shaking hands, sitting in public places, or even as health care workers, these antigens attempt to enter our bodies, without success – at first! The antigens sit on our clothing or on our skin just waiting for the right opportunity to assault us. This is one reason why regular and thorough washing of our bodies (and our clothing) is an excellent contribution to good health. In most medical facilities, their mantra is – the first line of defense is good hand washing!

Clean Fact – Hand washing is the first line of defense against germs and bacteria. Brisk hand washing for at least 20 seconds using soap and warm water will kill and remove most antigens.

Clean Fact – The HIV virus, as deadly as it is in the human body, is very unstable outside of the body. If a surface is contaminated by the AIDS virus, it can be decontaminated by using a Clorox solution. If intact skin comes in contact with the AIDS virus, simple soap and water with good hand washing technique is sufficient to kill the virus.

(In 2010, we learned from the local news that
scientists discovered HIV in a trash receptacle,
still alive and stable for at least 3 days)

Clean Fact – Nosocomial illnesses – illnesses that are acquired by patients during their hospital stay – most often occur due to failure of healthcare workers to observe hospital policies regarding good hand washing and other germ transmission preventive measures, especially before and after patient care). Many illnesses and diseases caused by contact organisms can be avoided by proper habits of cleanliness.

Examples of illnesses/diseases that are preventable with good handwashing and universal precautions: STDs, Hepatitis, TB, Colds, Flu, the list goes on!

Additional Benefits of Water

Hydrotherapy is one type of water therapy which is an excellent alternative remedy for many ills. To name a few, warm and cold compresses will help to alleviate sinus pain & congestion, headaches, and soreness or pain from arthritis or rheumatism. Hot steam treatments will help the body to purge toxins, and can help to relieve respiratory symptoms stemming from allergies, colds & flu and bronchitis or asthma. Steam is also a very useful beauty treatment for the face and skin.

Why is this important?

A Healthful Diet

Someone once said that we are what we eat, and it seems to be so true! We should learn to crave living foods that impart health, strength and vitality – while avoiding foods that weaken us. This means a diet consisting of plant-based foods is ideal to help us achieve optimal health. You might be surprised to find that the more often and regularly you eat healthy foods, the more you will begin to desire it. Simultaneously, you will begin to lose your desire for fast foods, meat products and processed foods.

- Bodies require wholesome food that provides the tools and materials needed for building a fine temple

- Overeating creates the need for extra storage space for whatever is not used by the body, thus creating obesity. Temperance is vital for health

- Balance is required in selecting foods for health and life. The materials you put into a house will determine the value of the house and the quality of it. Low quality, unhealthful foods may look appealing on the surface, but once the 'gloss' wears off, what do you think you'll see underneath?

- Eating should be a pleasurable experience, but the most important purpose is to promote health and life

I should be able to eat anything I want, right?
The answer is "yes". Of course, we all select the foods we want to eat based on our likes and dislikes, and sometimes for their health benefits. However, food plays a much more important role in your optimal health than you might imagine, so foods that impart vitality and strength are always the best choice.

Your body is self-healing, and when given the wholesome nutrition provided by nature, your body has the right materials needed to repair any damage, and help you to build a solid, stable temple. Begin your healing journey towards an organic, raw-vegetarian diet and you will soon begin to experience amazing results!

Even if this is not the type of food you are accustomed to eating, don't despair. You can set your own pace by adding one healthy food item to your diet at a time. As you practice eating healthfully, your body will begin to desire it more. Pretty soon, you will discover that you have discarded the unhealthful items from your life, and are making great strides towards your optimal health. And your body will love it!

It is possible to have health and healing even if you are not vegan-vegetarian. Naturally-bred, non-GMO, organic meat and poultry, added to a well-balanced diet with a wide variety of produce, will help you to enjoy a measure of health. Just remember that when we put dead foods into our bodies, it WILL have its detrimental effects, and will decelerate the healing process. Just remember that, the more closely we align ourselves with nature's diet, the easier it becomes to gain healing and reach a state of health and wellness.

All of us must determine the effects our food choices have on our health. Honestly assess your diet and decide if it could be better. For instance, think about how many of your favorite foods add pounds or inches to your mid-section, or dangerously raise your blood pressure. Then decide to make gradual changes as they are comfortable for you. It isn't about the opinions of others, and there are no diet police to make sure you don't slip up. When all is said and done, this whole topic of diet is about the type of materials you are selecting to build the type of temple **you** want to build… (remember your *recipe* and the *end result* you desire?)

If you would love to experience natural healing, then a plant-based, whole foods (vegan-vegetarian) diet is the best solution. Eat *LIVING* foods as was always intended for us – nature's foods that impart health, healing and life!

Why spend so much time on the subject of a Healthful Diet? Because…

… many people cringe at the thought of being vegetarian. I want to change your perception to one of excited anticipation

… many people have no control over what goes into their mouths. I want to help you regain control of your appetite

… the thought of having a plant-based diet is scarier than the reality of it. Your body will actually love it!

… I want to show you that it *can* be done; Once you've seen all of the benefits you've gained, you'll wish you had done it sooner

… so many diseases and illnesses begin with a poor diet. Likewise, natural health and healing begins with a well-balanced, healthy diet

… even if your transition to a vegan diet takes the next ten years, you will still reap the healing benefits during your journey

Those who choose to consume a raw diet should be careful to select fresh produce that is organic, without pesticides, non-radiated, non-GMO, and vine-ripened if you would gain the best benefits of a whole foods, natural diet. Make a wash solution of lemon juice and water, Apple Cider Vinegar (ACV) and water or an organic, non-toxic, store-bought solution. Soak produce for 2-3 minutes, then wash raw produce thoroughly to remove any foreign matter that might be still attached.

Activities to help establish Healthful Dietary Habits
Recommendations:

1. **If you must have meat** in your diet, check your local health food stores for meats that are organic, free from antibiotics, steroids & hormones, and that are non-GMO, and free-range (Avoid pond-bred fish) It may cost a bit more, but consider it an investment in your good health

2. **Treat yourself** to a meat entrée' meal 2-3 times per week until your meat cravings gradually diminish

3. **Regularly include** plenty of fresh fruit, vegetables, raw nuts and grains or grain products to your diet

4. **Eliminate pork** from your diet altogether. Using this animal food is one of the worst, most detrimental departures from a healthful diet for many reasons

5. **Ask at your local health food store** for suggestions on tasty meat substitutes and non-meat recipes

6. **Find healthful recipes** to make your vegetables more inviting and tasty

7. **If you have cravings** for unhealthy foods that you are accustomed to eating, try having a <u>small</u> amount to satisfy your cravings, then pay attention to your body's response to this food (*Learning your Wellness Language – Volume 2*). If you experience a positive response, then that particular food may not be as bad for you as you think. If you experience a negative response, decide for yourself when and how to eliminate that food from your life.

Remember: you are what you eat, and what you eat is always your choice!

Why is this important?

Herbal & Alternative Remedies

Between overeating, consuming all the wrong foods, overworking, losing sleep, being attacked by one germ or another, heredity and a host of other factors, we sometimes find ourselves facing a debilitating disease or illness despite our best efforts. This isn't the time to give it all up, but to realize that sometimes we just need a little extra 'healing help'.

When we are afflicted with any ailment, our body automatically begins the balancing and healing process. When our body's defense and repair system needs reinforcements, Herbal and Alternative Remedies offer the solutions that will soothe and heal without detrimental risks or side-effects.

Herbal & Alternative Remedies (natural remedies) can offer the needed assistance and bridge the gap between poor health and holistic healing.

The Good Thing about Herbs is that herbs are helpful without creating other health problems. With prescription drug medications, it is just the opposite. Instead of building up or healing the body, drugs "tear down", and this is indicated by what we all know as side-effects. You have probably noticed that every prescription drug has more than one side-effect. If you ask, most physicians will tell you that the side-effects are usually the lesser of two evils (Do you agree with that statement?). Many drugs will alleviate the symptoms of your disease or ailment, but in so doing, you will more than likely experience additional symptoms which will require additional treatment(s) and even more medication. Remember: <u>Drugs Do Not Cure!</u>

Another good thing about herbs is that you are not required to take herbs for the remainder of your life. Natural herbs are wonderfully useful in numerous ways: they are great for use in cooking, pest repellants or deodorizers, potpourri, alternative medicines, aromatherapy, and they have a decorative effect in gardens and flower arrangements. If we would adopt the God-given diet, we would not require drug medications, because the human body was designed to heal itself - given the right materials. Herbs do assist the body in its healing process and can be discontinued when the health concern has been addressed and remedied, unless you just like the way it tastes.

One more good thing about herbs (but definitely not the last) is that they are readily available, and you do not need a prescription (The supporters of pharmaceuticals have been attempting to gain control of the herbal industry for years). You can even grow, dry and use herbs on your own. You can try herbs without fear of harm, contrary to what many 'experts' are now saying. Just make sure you are educated about the herbs and their uses. Like poison ivy, some plants do possess certain properties that can potentially cause unpleasant reactions, so become knowledgeable about the plants you are using.

Natural Remedies have consistently proven effective for treating a multitude of health conditions. There are many people who have found true healing by using these 'old-home' remedies, and have also avoided the harmful side-effects caused or created by the use of pharmaceuticals and current medical treatments. However, the public trend towards utilizing natural remedies has also brought with it a few hindrances to effective treatment.

The general mindset seems to be that:

A. 'going natural' is simply a matter of replacing my drug medications with herbs
NOT!
B. it's better to suffer than to take medication
NOT!
C. I can have natural health and healing without following all the steps of the process
NOT!
D. natural remedies are the same as drug medication – one herb fits all
NOT!
E. sometimes we need to take drug medications
NOT!

This chapter on Herbal and Alternative remedies was written to elevate the general mindset from a level of fear and skepticism to one of trust and acceptance, to offer proven, reliable information regarding natural and alternative remedies in an effort to correct the many misconceptions that abound and to help those seeking to enjoy a natural, holistic lifestyle to successfully utilize these healing remedies.

Healing with Herbal & Alternative Remedies

Common Ailments and Helpful Herbs

Try to avoid asking the common question, "what can I take in place of my pills that is all natural?". It's actually best if you didn't think in terms of "what can I take to help this?" at all. Rather, ask yourself "what can I do to improve or obtain and maintain optimum health?"

What are Herbs? Herbs are simply fresh or dried plant parts

Just about every living plant has at least one medicinal property that can be used effectively to address several ailments. Most herbs can be used for several ailments with remarkable results, particularly if you are already practicing a healthy lifestyle. Because plants are living foods, we can benefit from their life-giving properties the most when they are consumed uncooked. When they are dried, these same properties are available for our health and healing. Every part of the plant has a purpose in the natural, holistic lifestyle. In essence, Herbal Remedies is about utilizing whole or natural food (plants) to heal whatever ails.

<u>A Few Rules for Using Herbs</u>

- When taking herbs for medicinal use, continue as directed by your naturopathic practitioner until the condition has been remedied. Then follow directions for discontinuing
- Use herbs that have been grown organically and away from high traffic areas
- You can easily grow your own window-sill herb garden at home. Use fresh herbs in raw salads, and fresh or dried for cooking
- Many herbs are now available in capsules, extracts, tea bags and bulk. Grow your own or Buy your organic herbs from trusted sources
- Consult with me, visit your local Natural Health Practitioner or take a class in Herbology to learn the proper usage of healing herbs *(to schedule a free consultation, visit: www.jclaresvnl.com)*

<u>Why is this important?</u>

*Stay connected with **jClare's Vibrant Natural Life** for upcoming courses and classes on Herbal Remedies!*
www.jclaresvnl.com

How to Make a Cup of Herbal Deliciousness!

1. Start with an 8 oz. cup and mesh strainer or tea ball
2. Add 1 teaspoon of your favorite herb to the strainer
3. Add ¼ teaspoon of Stevia leaves with the herb
4. Place the closed tea ball into your cup
5. Pour boiling water over the tea ball and cover with the saucer (this is steeping)
6. Allow your tea to steep for at least 5 minutes
7. You may use raw honey or Sugar-In-the-Raw instead of Stevia for a sweetener
8. Uncover your teacup, sit in your favorite rocking chair, sip, relax, enjoy!

A few Herb suggestions for Relaxing Tea Time

Sage	Chamomile
Cinnamon	Lemon/Ginger
Raspberry	Fennel/Ginger

Contact Your Naturopathic Consultant for more information on healing herbs

What are Alternative Remedies?

Alternative Remedies are various non-scientific, non-medical, healing modalities that utilize only those elements found in the natural world, and that pose no health risk to those seeking natural healing. Many in the scientific/medical community view Alternative Remedies as fraudulent or quackery because their effectiveness cannot be proven scientifically. However, these methods have been used effectively when traditional medical treatments have proven ineffective or have resulted in a worsened condition. Alternative healing practices often employ stimulation or manipulation of the pressure points, the nerves and energy centers (chakras), the spine and other bones & muscles. Plus, they require a measure of faith and belief, along with a positive mental attitude, thus presenting a more holistic approach to health and healing.

Because alternative practices are generally unregulated, this type of healing seems more open to frauds and quacks, which is a good reason for caution. But throughout the years, there have also been cases of fraud and malpractice in traditional medicine. Therefore, it is always wise to do your homework and become proactive in all of your health decisions regarding treatments and therapies. Get a second or even a third opinion and pay close attention to patient reviews regarding particular medical professionals. Research any health practitioner, whether traditional or alternative. Speak with previous clients, get all the information you can about any type of new therapy, and try to understand the mechanism of action of any treatment. Be wise in your selection of health care providers.

With all of the negativity surrounding Alternative Remedies, why bother? Well, I figure if it doesn't harm you in any way, and can offer numerous benefits, what do you have to lose? Miraculous healings that defy rhyme and reason have been documented since biblical times, and for people of faith, that's important. Let's take a look at the pros and cons of Alternative Remedies, and compare that to traditional medicine...

The Pros – Alternative Remedies:

- are generally non-invasive (Acupuncture is one exception)
- are holistic – (healing to mind, body & spirit altogether) – the person does not need to sacrifice the health of one part for healing to occur in another
- allow you to actively engage and express your personal spiritual beliefs
- generally, have no negative side-effects
- are creative as opposed to being destructive
- are harmonious with nature
- utilize natural healing resources
- tend to focus first on spiritual and mental healing which results in physical healing
- are offered by a largely unregulated, unlicensed community – anyone with the gifts, skills and talents can offer their services
- are not standardized, therefore are more open & receptive to individual gifts and talents and their place in healing

The Cons – Alternative Remedies:

- are offered by a largely unregulated, unlicensed community – any fraud or quack can do it
- are not standardized, therefore offers no consistency from one practitioner to another
- have a mechanism of action that cannot be explained nor proven scientifically
- may have origins stemming from the supernatural, metaphysics and other scary mystical stuff

A Few Alternative Remedies

Many Alternative Remedies and therapies are safe and reliable healing modalities, yet there are also a few that you might want to avoid. Do not become overly eager to place the responsibility of your health and wellness upon anyone else. Don't be governed by ignorance, fear or prejudice. Do base your decisions on study, research and knowledge, maintaining a sense of the value of your personal beliefs & preferences regarding what is best for your health. Be open to new ideas of health and healing, have a positive mentality, and allow your faith to expand in a positive, holistic direction.

I've listed a few Alternative therapies that I believe are worth checking out. Do your research and you might be surprised that one or more of these offer just what you've been looking for.

Iridology
Acupressure
Massage Therapy
Energy Therapies (Reiki)
Herbology
Holistic Health
Mind-Body Medicine
Meditation
Hydrotherapy
Chiropractic
Acupuncture
Homeopathy
Tai Chi

<u>**Why is this important?**</u>

Let's recap!

The God Connection

Meditation: A Healthy Mind & Emotions

Exercise & Recreation

Relaxation & Restful Sleep

Sunshine & Fresh Air

Proper Elimination

Pure Water

A Healthful Diet

Herbal & Alternative Remedies

Revealing the Mysteries of Natural Healing has introduced to you an outline of the guidelines that must be in place for natural healing to begin. It is vital to your holistic health and healing that you make these guidelines key factors in your lifestyle choices. A balanced combination of these guidelines is necessary for creating your amazing, natural, holistic, healthy lifestyle. But balancing these is not a one-size-fits-all situation, and your optimum health and healing has just begun. To create your own, unique, healthy balance, you must now learn to understand and utilize your wellness language.

As you incorporate these natural healing guidelines into your life, you will begin to notice your body responding in new and different ways – some expected, and a few possibly a little uncomfortable. You are beginning to hear and recognize *Your Wellness Language*, which is essential for you to understand if you wish to attain and maintain your personal healthy balance. Everyone has a personal healthy balance, and this internal communications system will show you the best means of reaching yours. When you learn to trust your wellness language, you are definitely on the path that leads you to optimal, holistic health and wellness!

Look for the additional volumes of

Healing Through Nature's Eyes

and companion workbooks:

Volume 1 – Revealing the Mysteries of Natural Healing
Volume 2 – Learning Your Wellness Language
Volume 3 – Eloquence in Nature's Healing Language

Visit:

j Clare's Vibrant Natural Life

www.jclaresvnl.com

www.ingramcontent.com/pod-product-compliance
Lightning Source LLC
Chambersburg PA
CBHW060816290526
45792CB00005BB/1676